Units, Symbols, and

A Guide for Authors and Editors in

Units, Symbols, and Abbreviations

A Guide for Authors and Editors in Medicine and Related Sciences

Sixth Edition

D N Baron MA, MD, DSc, FRCP, FRCPath
H McKenzie Clarke MA, MSc

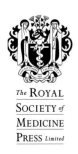

The ROYAL
SOCIETY *of*
MEDICINE
PRESS *Limited*

© 2008 Royal Society of Medicine Press Ltd

Published by the Royal Society of Medicine Press Ltd
1 Wimpole Street, London W1G 0AE, UK
Tel: +44 (0)20 7290 2921
Fax: +44 (0)20 7290 2929
Email: publishing@rsm.ac.uk
Website: www.rsmpress.co.uk

First edition 1971
Revised 1972
Reprinted 1975
Third edition 1977
Fourth edition 1988
Fifth edition 1994

The Royal Society of Medicine Press has no responsibility for the reliability or accuracy of URLs for the external or third-party websites cited in this publication and therefore cannot guarantee their content is, or will remain, accurate or relevant. 10 0054 8003 36

The rights of D N Baron and H McKenzie Clarke to be identified as authors of this work have been asserted by them in accordance with the Copyright, Designs and Patents Act, 1988.

British Library Cataloguing in Publication Data
A catalogue record for this book is available from the British Library

ISBN 978-1-85315-624-3

Distribution in Europe and Rest of World:
Marston Book Services Ltd
PO Box 269
Abingdon
Oxon OX14 4YN, UK
Tel: +44 (0)1235 465500
Fax: +44 (0)1235 465555
Email: direct.order@marston.co.uk

Distribution in the USA and Canada:
Royal Society of Medicine Press Ltd
c/o BookMasters Inc
30 Amberwood Parkway
Ashland, OH 44805, USA
Tel: +1 800 247 6553/+1 800 266 5564
Fax: +1 419 281 6883
Email: orders@bookmasters.com

Distribution in Australia and New Zealand:
Elsevier Australia
30–52 Smidmore Street
Marrickville NSW 2204, Australia
Tel: +61 2 9517 8999
Fax: +61 2 9517 2249
Email: service@elsevier.com.au

Typeset by Phoenix Photosetting, Chatham, Kent
Printed in Europe by the Alden Group, Oxford

Contents

Preface

As new recommendations continue to be made on the International System of Units (SI), and on terminology and practice used in medical and biological science by national and international organizations, so new symbols, abbreviations, and conventions come into use.

The fifth edition of *Units, Symbols, and Abbreviations* (1994) was published 14 years ago, and it was decided that there were sufficient new developments and changes in this area to warrant a new edition, with an additional author. The general layout of the last edition has been retained, but the great change since that edition has been the introduction of electronic media and their continuing substitution for paper texts [*AD 2020: 'Mummy, what's a book?'*]. This is reflected in this edition by the fact that many of the sources for conventions for units and guidelines on terminology are now on websites instead of or in addition to printed material.

Chapter 1 provides a brief description of the units of the SI and gives some guidance on how numbers and unit symbols should be represented in print. Chapter 2 outlines the principles for forming symbols and abbreviations, with comments on conventions; this is followed by a fully referenced general listing. In Chapter 3, the Vancouver and Harvard referencing systems are discussed, and digital object identifiers are briefly described. In Chapter 4, on proof correction, the layout has been simplified, and account is taken of recent recommendations by the British Standards Institution.

The authors would like to thank Ms Alison Campbell, Ms Hannah Wessely, and the editorial team at the Royal Society of Medicine Press for their help. Thanks are also due to the libraries of the British Medical Association, the Royal Free Hospital School of Medicine, and the Royal Society of Medicine for their support. Our aim has been to set out national and international standard practice, and we hope that authors, editors, and publishers will continue to find this publication useful. Comments and suggestions for future editions are welcome and should be sent to us, c/o Royal Society of Medicine Press, 1 Wimpole Street, London W1G 0AE.

DNB
HMC

1 | Units

The International System of Units (Système International d'Unités: SI) was established in 1960 by the General Conference on Weights and Measures (Conférence Générale des Poids et Mesures: CGPM). Together with the International Committee for Weights and Measures (Comité International des Poids et Mesures: CIPM) and the International Bureau of Weights and Measures (Bureau International des Poids et Mesures: BIPM), the CGPM is also responsible for maintaining and developing the SI. Further details about the work of these bodies can be found on their respective web pages:

www.bipm.org/en/convention/cgpm

www.bipm.org/en/committees/cipm

www.bipm.org/en/bipm

An account of the historical development of the SI and a list of the relevant decisions of the CGPM and CIPM regarding definitions of units and conventions can be found in the *SI Brochure*, 8th edition, which is available at www.bipm.org/en/si/si_brochure.

The present chapter provides a brief description of the units of the SI; a complete presentation, with a general background discussion on establishing a system of units, is given in the *SI Brochure*, cited above. The final section of the chapter gives some guidance on how numbers and unit symbols should be represented in print.

SI base units

There are seven base quantities, with corresponding units, in the SI: length (metre), mass (kilogram), time (second), electric current (ampere), thermodynamic temperature (kelvin), amount of substance (mole), and luminous intensity (candela). The definitions of these base units are given in Table 1.1.

SI derived units

Derived units are formed from products of powers (positive or negative) of the base units (see pages 8 and 9 for details of how these should be represented). The SI is a *coherent* system of units; that is, equations between numerical values of quantities have exactly the same form as the corresponding equations between the quantities themselves. In a coherent system, no numerical factor other than 1 ever occurs in the expressions for the derived units in terms of the base units. Thus, for example, the unit of velocity is the metre per second ($m\ s^{-1}$) and the unit of density is the kilogram per cubic metre ($kg\ m^{-3}$). Certain derived units have their own names and symbols: these are shown in Table 1.2. Note that these derived units may be expressed in terms of each other as well as in terms of the base units.

Table 1.1 SI base quantities, units, and definitions

Base quantity	Unit name	Unit symbol
Length	metre	m
Mass	kilogram	kg
Time, duration	second	s
Electric current	ampere	A
Thermodynamic temperature	kelvin	K
Amount of substance	mole	mol
Luminous intensity	candela	cd

Definition of unit

The metre is the length of the path travelled by light in vacuum during a time interval of 1/299 792 458 of a second[a]

The kilogram is the unit of mass; it is equal to the mass of the international prototype of the kilogram[b]

The second is the duration of 9 192 631 770 periods of the radiation corresponding to the transition between the two hyperfine levels of the ground state of the caesium-133 atom[c]

The ampere is that constant current which, if maintained in two straight parallel conductors of infinite length, of negligible circular cross-section, and placed 1 metre apart in vacuum, would produce between these conductors a force equal to 2×10^{-7} newton per metre of length

The kelvin, unit of thermodynamic temperature, is the fraction 1/273.16 of the thermodynamic temperature of the triple point of water[d]

1. The mole is the amount of substance in a system that contains as many entities as there are atoms in 0.012 kilogram of carbon-12[e]
2. When the mole is used, the elementary entities must be specified and may be atoms, molecules, ions, electrons, other particles, or specified groups of such particles

The candela is the luminous intensity, in a given direction, of a source that emits monochromatic radiation of frequency 540×10^{12} hertz and that has a radiant intensity in that direction of 1/683 watt per steradian

[a]The speed of light in vacuum is *defined* as exactly 299 792 458 metres per second.
[b]It should be noted that the kilogram is the only one of the SI base units that is still defined in terms of a physical artefact, leading to problems concerning the stability of that artefact and thus of the unit itself. Research is therefore underway to find a method of redefining the kilogram in terms of a fixed value of a fundamental or atomic constant (Planck's constant or Avogadro's constant), similar to the way in which the metre is now defined in terms of the speed of light. (Consideration is also being given to redefining the ampere, the kelvin, and the mole in terms of fixed values of fundamental constants.)
[c]This definition refers to a caesium atom at rest at a temperature of 0 K (i.e. unperturbed by black body radiation).
[d]Of an exactly specified isotopic composition.
[e]Unbound carbon-12 atoms, at rest and in their ground state.

Table 1.2 SI derived units with special names and symbols

Quantity	Unit name	Unit symbol	In terms of other SI units	In terms of SI base units	Notes
Absorbed dose, specific energy (imparted), kerma	gray	Gy	$J\,kg^{-1}$	$m^2\,s^{-2}$	*a*
Activity referred to a radionuclide	becquerel	Bq		s^{-1}	*a, b*
Capacitance	farad	F	$C\,V^{-1}$	$A^2\,m^{-2}\,kg^{-1}\,s^4$	
Catalytic activity	katal	kat		$mol\,s^{-1}$	*a*
Celsius temperature	degree Celsius	°C		K	*c*
Dose equivalent (ambient, directional, or personal)	sievert	Sv	$J\,kg^{-1}$	$m^2\,s^{-2}$	*a*
Electric charge, amount of electricity	coulomb	C		A s	
Electric conductance	siemens	S	$A\,V^{-1}$	$A^2\,m^{-2}\,kg^{-1}\,s^3$	
Electric potential difference, electromotive force	volt	V	$W\,A^{-1}$	$m^2\,kg\,s^{-3}\,A^{-1}$	
Electric resistance	ohm	Ω	$V\,A^{-1}$	$m^2\,kg\,s^{-3}\,A^{-2}$	
Energy, work, amount of heat	joule	J	N m	$m^2\,kg\,s^{-2}$	
Force	newton	N		$m\,kg\,s^{-2}$	
Frequency	hertz	Hz		s^{-1}	*b*
Illuminance	lux	lx	$lm\,m^{-2}$	$cd\,m^{-2}$	
Inductance	henry	H	$Wb\,A^{-1}$	$m^2\,kg\,s^{-2}\,A^{-2}$	
Luminous flux	lumen	lm	cd sr	cd	
Magnetic flux	weber	Wb	V s	$m^2\,kg\,s^{-2}\,A^{-1}$	

4

Table 1.2 SI derived units with special names and symbols *(continued)*

Quantity	Unit name	Unit symbol	In terms of other SI units	In terms of SI base units	Notes
Magnetic flux density	tesla	T	Wb m^{-2}	kg s^{-2} A^{-1}	
Plane angle	radian	rad	1	m m^{-1}	d
Power, radiant flux	watt	W	J s^{-1}	kg m^2 s^{-3}	
Pressure, stress	pascal	Pa	N m^{-2}	kg m^{-1} s^{-2}	
Solid angle	steradian	sr	1	m^2 m^{-2}	d

[a]These quantities have been admitted specifically for reasons of safeguarding human health.
[b]The hertz is the name for the inverse second in the general context of periodic phenomena; the becquerel is the name used specifically in the context of stochastic activity related to a radionuclide.
[c]The degree Celsius is the special name for the kelvin when stating Celsius temperatures. Since the degree Celsius and the kelvin are of equal magnitude, a temperature difference or temperature interval has the same numerical value when expressed in either unit.
[d]The radian and steradian can be considered as special names for the number 1 that may be incorporated in derived units to convey information about the quantity concerned (directional distributions in two and three dimensions, respectively). The radian is the plane angle subtended at the centre of a circle by an arc equal in length to the radius. The steradian is the solid angle subtended at the centre of a sphere by an area of the surface equal to the square of the length of the radius.

SI prefixes

Decimal multiples (from 10^1 to 10^{24}) and submultiples (from 10^{-1} to 10^{-24}) of SI units may be represented by prefixes. The names of these prefixes and the corresponding symbols are given in Table 1.3.

A number of points should be noted with regard to the use of these prefixes:

- Prefix names must be closed up, without spacing or hyphenation, to unit names: for example microsecond and kilopascal.

- Prefix symbols must also be closed up to unit symbols: for example μs and kPa.

- A prefix symbol must always be followed *directly* by a unit symbol: thus, for example, k/m^3 is unacceptable as an alternative to 10^3 m^{-3} or 10^3/m^3, and μ must not be used as shorthand for μm.

- An exponent used with a prefixed unit refers to the entire unit: thus, mm^3 means 1 cubic millimetre, not 10^{-3} cubic metres.

- Multiple prefixes and prefix symbols must not be used: for example, μmm is not acceptable as an alternative to nm.

Table 1.3 Prefixes for SI units

Factor	Prefix	Symbol	Factor	Prefix	Symbol
10^{-1}	deci	d	10^{1}	deca	da
10^{-2}	centi	c	10^{2}	hecto	h
10^{-3}	milli	m	10^{3}	kilo	k
10^{-6}	micro	μ	10^{6}	mega	M
10^{-9}	nano	n	10^{9}	giga	G
10^{-12}	pico	p	10^{12}	tera	T
10^{-15}	femto	f	10^{15}	peta	P
10^{-18}	atto	a	10^{18}	exa	E
10^{-21}	zepto	z	10^{21}	zetta	Z
10^{-24}	yocto	y	10^{24}	yotta	Y

- For historical reasons, the kilogram, although an SI base unit, incorporates a prefix in both its name and its symbol. Therefore, names and symbols for decimal multiples and submultiples of the unit of mass are formed by attaching prefixes and prefix symbols to the name 'gram' and the symbol 'g', even though the gram is not an SI base unit: for example, 10^{-6} kg is written as mg (not μkg) and, of course, 10^{-3} kg as g (not mkg).

Non-SI units

Units defined exactly in terms of SI units
There are some units that, although they are not part of the SI, are accepted for use with the SI because of their widespread use in everyday life. These units, which are shown in Table 1.4, are defined exactly in terms of SI units.

Units with experimentally determined values
In some scientific fields, there are certain advantages in using particular non-SI units that are related to fundamental constants (electron mass and charge, etc.), the values of which in terms of SI units must be determined experimentally. Most of these units are used specifically in high-energy physics, atomic physics, and quantum chemistry, and will not be given here. However, there are three that are relevant to biomedical sciences and are accepted for use with the SI; they are shown in Table 1.5.

Units originating from the CGS and CGS–Gaussian systems
The CGS system of units is formulated in terms of the centimetre, gram, and second as base units of length, mass, and time. There is no independent base unit for electrical and magnetic quantities corresponding to the ampere in the SI; instead, electrical and magnetic units are derived from those for length, mass, and time in various ways (involving fractional powers of

Table 1.4 Non-SI units accepted for use with the SI with values defined exactly in terms of SI units

Quantity	Unit name	Unit symbol	Value in SI units[a]
Time	minute	min	60 s
	hour	h	3600 s
	day	d	86 400 s
Plane angle	degree	°	$(\pi/180)$ rad
	minute	′	$(\pi/10\ 800)$ rad
	second (arcsecond)	″	$(\pi/648\ 000)$ rad
Area (land)	hectare	ha	$1\ hm^2 = 10^4\ m^2$
Volume	litre[b]	L, l	$1\ dm^3 = 10^3\ cm^3 = 10^{-3}\ m^3$
Mass	tonne ('metric ton')	t	$10^3\ kg$

[a]These values constitute *definitions* and are therefore exact.
[b]Exceptionally, two symbols are acceptable for the litre, with the newer symbol L having been introduced to avoid possible confusion with the number 1. It should be noted that an earlier definition of the litre (leading to a value of 1.000 028 dm^3) has been replaced by the above definition. Furthermore, it is recommended that the litre (and millilitre, etc.) should not be used to give the results of highly accurate volume measurements.

Table 1.5 Non-SI units accepted for use with the SI the values of which must be obtained experimentally

Quantity	Unit name	Unit symbol	Value in SI units[a,b]
Energy	electronvolt[c]	eV	$1.602\ 176\ 487\ (40) \times 10^{-19}$ J
Mass	dalton[d]	Da	$1.660\ 538\ 782\ (83) \times 10^{-27}$ kg
	unified atomic mass unit[d]	u	1 u = 1 Da

[a]Taken from Mohr PJ, Taylor BN, Newell DB. The 2006 CODATA Recommended Values of the Fundamental Physical Constants (Web Version 5.0). Gaithersburg, MD: National Institute of Standards and Technology, 2007. Available at physics.nist.gov/constants and arxiv.org/abs/0801.0028.
[b]The standard uncertainty in the last two digits is given in parentheses.
[c]Defined as the kinetic energy acquired by an electron in passing through a potential difference of 1 V in vacuum. The electronvolt is often used in combination with SI prefixes (keV, etc.).
[d]These are alternative names for the same unit, which is equal to $\frac{1}{12}$ the mass of a free carbon-12 atom, at rest in its ground state. The dalton is often used in combination with SI prefixes, especially when giving the masses of large molecules in kilodaltons (kDa).

these latter units), leading to the CGS–electrostatic, CGS–electromagnetic, and CGS–Gaussian systems. These systems (especially the CGS–Gaussian) have advantages in certain areas of physics, including some of relevance to biomedical sciences, and are often encountered in the older literature. Therefore, although the use of such units with the SI is not encouraged, those that have been given special names are listed in Table 1.6.

Table 1.6 Non-SI units originating from the CGS and CGS–Gaussian systems

Quantity	Unit name	Unit symbol	Value in SI units
Energy	erg	erg	10^{-7} J
Force	dyne	dyn	10^{-5} N
Illuminance	phot	ph	10^{4} lx
Luminance	stilb	sb	10^{4} cd m^{-2}
Magnetic field	oersted	Oe	$[(10^{3}/4\pi)$ A m^{-1} = $(250/\pi)$ A m$^{-1}]^{a}$
Magnetic flux	maxwell	Mx	$[10^{-8}$ Wb$]^{a}$
Magnetic flux density	gauss	G	$[10^{-4}$ T$]^{a}$
Viscosity:			
dynamic	poise	P	0.1 Pa s
kinematic	stokes	St	10^{-4} m^{2} s^{-1}

[a]In the GGS–Gaussian system, the definitions of electrical and magnetic quantities differ from those in the SI. Therefore, strictly speaking, values of such quantities in the two systems cannot be directly compared; rather, for example, a magnetic field *as defined in the CGS–Gaussian system* with a value of 1 Oe *corresponds* to a magnetic field *as defined in the SI* with a value of $(250/\pi)$ A m^{-1}.

Other non-SI units

Many other non-SI units have been used in the past or are now used only in particular fields or particular countries (e.g. Imperial Units in the UK and US Customary Units in the USA). They should not be used with the SI; if values of quantities are quoted in these units, the SI equivalent must also be given. Some such units are given in Chapter 2; a comprehensive list, together with conversion factors to SI units, is given in Appendix B of Taylor BN. *Guide for the Use of the International System of Units (SI). NIST Special Publication 811.* Gaithersburg, MD: National Institute of Standards and Technology, 1995. Available at physics.nist.gov/Pubs/SP811.

Numbers and unit symbols

Numbers

Integers

In integers of more than four digits, the digits should be split into groups of three, from right to left, separated by thin spaces. This should be done for four-digit integers only if they are in a table column that also contains larger integers. Note that, to avoid possible confusion with the widespread use internationally of the comma to represent the decimal marker, the groups of digits must *not* be separated by commas.

Examples:

1 328 765	*not*	1328765 or 1,328,765
2395	*not*	2,395 or (except in tables) 2 395

8

Decimal numbers

For the decimal marker, the CGPM sanctions the use of either the point on the line or the comma. However, in English-language publications, the point is almost universally used. Note that for decimal numbers less than 1, the point must always be preceded by a zero. For clarity, digits to the right of the decimal marker may be split similarly to those to the left.

Examples:

0.512   *not*   .512

19.769 266 91   *or*   19.76926691

Multiplication

In scientific (exponential) notation for numbers, multiplication should be indicated by a multiplication sign rather than a raised point.

Example:

4.2982×10^{-5} *not* $4.2982 \cdot 10^{-5}$

Unit symbols

Unit symbols should be in roman (upright) type. A symbol should be separated from a preceding number by a thin space, not closed up.

Symbols for derived units

Products of unit symbols may be represented by either a thin space or a raised point. Symbols must not be closed up to one another, because of the risk of confusion between units and prefixes.

Examples:

N m	*or*	N·m	*not*	Nm
kg m^2	*or*	kg·m^2	*not*	kgm^2

Quotients of unit symbols may be represented either using a solidus or negative exponents. When the solidus is used, parentheses must be inserted where necessary to avoid possible ambiguity.

Examples:

m s^{-1}	*or*	m·s^{-1}	*or*	m/s		*not*	ms^{-1}
W m^{-2}	*or*	W·m^{-2}	*or*	W/m^2		*not*	Wm^{-2}
J mol^{-1} K^{-1}	*or*	J·mol^{-1}·K^{-1}	*or*	J/(mol K)	*or* J/(mol·K)	*not*	J/mol/K

2 | Symbols and nomenclature

Principles for forming symbols and abbreviations

The symbols, abbreviations, and conventions in the following list of recommendations are based upon current practice in British and international journals as shown in their Instructions to Authors and upon recommendations by relevant specialist societies, with the advice of expert colleagues.

The task of a codifier is not easy. Ideally, there is a firm internationally based ruling accepted by the appropriate national bodies – as in the case of the SI units described in Chapter 1. Thus, 'kg' is the universally accepted symbol for kilogram(s): any use of 'Kg', 'kgs', or 'kGm', for example, is *wrong*. Often, custom and convention have led to a widely, although not universally, accepted usage: an example is the use in biomedical sciences of P to denote partial pressure – the use of p is not wrong, but could lead to confusion with p as in pH. In the following list, when there is no uniformity, a recommendation is made that is most consistent with other accepted usage.

Accepted current practice for symbols and nomenclature
The following principles should be adhered to:

- **Physical quantities**   These are normally represented by single letters of the Latin or Greek alphabet, in italic (sloping) type, without full stops: for example volume, V; density, ρ.

- **Units** (see also Chapter 1)   These are normally represented by one or more letters of the Latin or Greek alphabet, in upright (roman) type, without full stops: for example metre, m; micromole, μmol. Symbols for units are usually in lower case, unless the unit is named after a person: for example joule, J. A notable exception is the symbol for litre: L is now an acceptable alternative to l because of the possible confusion of the latter with the number 1 in many typefaces (see Table 1.4).

- **Chemical substances**   Chemical elements are denoted by one or two Latin letters in upright type, without a full stop (the first letter is always a capital, the second always lower case). Abbreviations for chemical compounds are usually in upright capital letters from the Latin alphabet, without full stops: for example adenosine $5'$-triphosphate, ATP. A similar convention is applied to hormones, enzymes, cytokines, etc., with the abbreviation sometimes also including a number: for example follicle-stimulating hormone, FSH; creatine kinase, CK; erythropoietin, EPO. Greek letters, lower case letters, and numbers may also be used: for example interferon-α, INF-α; acetylcholine, ACh; interleukin-6, IL-6.

- **Species, including microorganisms**   The systematic names (of taxonomic categories) are normally in upper and lower case italic type (with a capital only in the generic component) when used for identification (e.g. *Staphylococcus aureus*) and in lower case upright type when used generally (e.g. the staphylococci or a staphylococcal infection).

Note that the names of taxonomic ranks higher than genus (i.e. family, . . ., domain) should be in upper and lower case roman type (e.g. family Enterobacteriaceae, order Enterobacteriales).

- **Genes** Gene symbols are in italic type; the use of capitalization varies between organisms.

Recommendations for abbreviations

- **Symbols** are international and cross-disciplinary, and so should be used whenever possible, especially in equations.

- **Abbreviations** (or **contractions**) are not necessarily international, as they may vary with language. Their purpose is to save space in tables, figures, etc., or when the same word occurs many times in the text of an article, book, or thesis. Their use in equations should be limited – symbols should preferably be employed (defined, if necessary, for a specific equation). All abbreviations must be defined at first mention unless likely to be familiar to most readers (many journals provide, in their Instructions to Authors, lists of abbreviations that need not be spelt out). Overuse of less familiar abbreviations can be a hindrance to foreign language readers and to interdisciplinary communication.

- Abbreviations for words in common use that are part of the word are normally in lower case upright type, ending with a full stop unless the abbreviation retains the final letter of the original word: for example, conc., concentrated; concn, concentration. The full stop is always omitted if the abbreviation is used as a subscript or superscript.

- Scientific and medical abbreviations that are combinations of initial letters are usually now in upper case upright type, without full stops: for example, CSF, cerebrospinal fluid; ECG, electrocardiogram; NMR, nuclear magnetic resonance. There are some exceptions: for example, f.p., freezing point; IV or i.v., intravenous.

- Abbreviations for measured physical quantities that may be followed by a number and a unit are normally in upper case upright type, without full stops: for example FEV, forced expiratory volume (e.g. FEV in 1 s, $FEV_1 = 3.6$ L).

Symbols, abbreviations, and conventions

The selection of items for this list, although necessarily arbitrary, is intended to include the terms most widely used in medicine and related sciences. The principles described above are followed as far as possible. It should be noted that conventions in other fields (e.g. high-energy physics and engineering) may sometimes be different. Further details of terminology in particular areas of biomedical science may be found in the sources listed in the references at the end of this list.

Symbols for chemical elements are not included here – these are widely available. Abbreviations for names of diseases, for physical signs and symptoms, and for names of drugs have also been excluded, as these are often local or not widely accepted.

The italicized words in the recommendations have the following meanings:

use	this is the recommended usage
or	there is at present no firm recommendation or usage

| *preferred* | it is hoped that the preferred alternative will become universal, but the non-preferred alternative will not cause confusion |
| *avoid/not* | this should never be used, as it is not consistent with established international terminology or is likely to cause confusion |

Some of the conversion factors in this list are approximate (indicated by $\approx$ rather than =); exact values can be found in Appendix B of Taylor BN. *Guide for the Use of the International System of Units (SI). NIST Special Publication 811.* Gaithersburg, MD: National Institute of Standards and Technology, 1995. Available at physics.nist.gov/Pubs/SP811.

about (numerically)		*preferred to c. (circa)* *avoid* ~ (as this can mean an energy-rich bond)
absolute	abs.	
absorbance	A	*preferred to* internal transmission density D_i
absorbed dose (ionizing radiation)	D	
absorption coefficient:		
molar	ε	*preferred to* absorptivity
specific	a	
acceleration	a	
acceleration due to gravity	g	for centrifugal conditions
acetylcholine	ACh	
acid-fast bacillus	AFB	
activated clotting time	ACT	
activated partial thromboplastin time	APTT *or* aPTT	
activity:		
nuclear physics	A	
physical chemistry	a	
adenine	A	
adenosine	A	deoxyadenosine: dA
adenosine 5′-monophosphate	AMP	
5′-diphosphate	ADP	
5′-triphosphate	ATP	
cyclic 3′:5′-monophosphate	cAMP	

adrenocorticotropic (adrenocorticotrophic) hormone	ACTH	*or* corticotropin (corticotrophin); see '-trophic/-trophin'
alanine	Ala, A	
alanine transaminase (aminotransferase)	ALT	
alcohol		*use* ethanol, methanol, etc., unless generically
alcohol- and acid-fast bacillus	AAFB	
α-fetoprotein	AFP	
alternating current	AC *or* a.c.	
alveolar	A	as suffix or subscript
alveolar minute ventilation	$\dot{V}_A$	
amino acids		see Refs 1, 2; *use* three-letter symbols in text; one-letter symbols may be used in sequences
amount of substance	n	unit: mole
analysis of variance (statistics)	ANOVA	
analytical standard of reagent purity	AR	
anatomical nomenclature		see Ref 3
angiotensin	Ang	
angiotensin-converting enzyme	ACE	
ångström	Å	*avoid*; *use* SI units (1 Å = 10^{-10} m = 0.1 nm)
angular velocity	ω	ω is also used for circular frequency (pulsatance)
anhydrous	anhyd.	
animals (experimental)		quote full binomial name at first mention (see Refs 4–6)
ante meridiem	a.m.	24-hour clock *preferred*
anterior	ant.	
antibody monoclonal	Ab mAb	

antidiuretic hormone (arginine vasopressin)	ADH	
antigen	Ag	
cluster of differentiation	CD	CD1, etc.
antigen-presenting cell	APC	
antineutrophil cytoplasmic antibody	ANCA	
cytoplasmic	c-ANCA *or* cANCA	
perinuclear	p-ANCA *or* pANCA	
antinuclear antibody	ANA	
antithrombin III	ATIII	antithrombin III is frequently referred to as simply antithrombin
approximately	approx.	
approximately equals	≈	*avoid* ~ (see 'about')
aqueous	aq.	
arabinose	Ara	
area	A	
area under the curve (of concentration vs time)	AUC	
arginine	Arg, R	
arginine vasopressin (antidiuretic hormone)	AVP	
arterial	a	particularly as suffix or subscript
arterial blood gases	ABG	
arteriovenous	a-v	
ascorbic acid		vitamin C *preferred* for consideration of biological activity
asparagine	Asn, N	
aspartate transaminase (aminotransferase)	AST	
aspartic acid	Asp, D	
atmosphere (standard)	atm	*avoid*; *use* kilopascal (1 atm = 101.325 kPa)
atmospheric	atm.	
atomic mass	m_a	

15

atomic mass unit (unified)	u	as $m_a(^{12}C)/12$; or use dalton; see Table 1.5
atomic weight	at. wt	relative atomic mass A_r (i.e. referred to the unit, u, which is $\frac{1}{12}$ the mass of the ^{12}C atom) is *preferred*
atrial natriuretic factor/peptide	ANF/ANP	
atrioventricular	AV	
average	av.	
bacterial artificial chromosome	BAC	
bacterial nomenclature		see Refs 7, 8; genus and species names should be in italic type, but when the genus name is used in a general sense, it should be in roman type without initial capital – e.g. *Staphylococcus aureus*, but staphylococci/staphylococcal
bar	bar	special name for 10^5 Pa (1 bar is used as the standard pressure for tabulating all thermodynamic data); *avoid* mb for millibar (1 mbar = 100 Pa);
basal metabolic rate	BMR	
base-pair	bp	
beats per minute	beats/min *or* bpm *or* b.p.m.	
billion		*avoid* in scientific writing (although in common usage for a thousand million); *use* appropriate power of 10 or SI prefix (see Table 1.3)
biochemical terminology and nomenclature		see Refs 1, 2
blood (e.g. laboratory reporting)	B	e.g. B-erythrocyte, diameter (mean) = 7.4 μm
blood groups		see Refs 9–11
blood pressure	BP	*preferably* give values in kPa, as well as mmHg (the clinical usage), in scientific writing
blood urea nitrogen (US only)	BUN	blood urea (in mmol/L) is *preferred*
body mass index	BMI	

boiling point	b.p.	*preferred to* bp
botanical nomenclature		see Ref 12
bovine serum albumin	BSA	
British National Formulary	BNF	give edition and date
British Pharmaceutical Codex	BPC	give edition and date
British Pharmacopoeia	BP	give edition and date
bulk modulus, modulus of compression	K	
calciferol		ergocalciferol is vitamin D_2, cholecalciferol is vitamin D_3; vitamin D is generic descriptor for biological activity
calciferol derivatives		e.g. 1,25-dihydroxycholecalciferol: $1,25\text{-}(OH)_2D_3$
calculated	calc.	
calorie (general)		*use* energy (e.g. low-energy diet)
calorie (unit of energy)	cal	may be used only in nutrition – otherwise *avoid*; *use* joule (1 cal = 4.184 J); do *not* use Calorie (Cal) as a synonym for kilocalorie (kcal)
capacitance	C	
capillary	c	particularly as a subscript
carbon: chain length position	e.g. C_{17} e.g. C-17	
carbon dioxide output	$\dot{V}_{CO_2}$	
carcinoembryonic antigen	CEA	
cardiac frequency	f_c	in beats/min
cardiac output	$\dot{Q}_t$ *or* CO	
cardiovascular magnetic resonance	CMR	
centigrade		*avoid*; *use* Celsius
centimetre of water (pressure)	cmH_2O	*use only* when measured manometrically; give SI equivalent in scientific writing (1 cmH_2O = 98.067 Pa)

centimorgan	cM	1% of crossovers
central nervous system	CNS	
central venous pressure	CVP	
centrifugal conditions		see Ref 1
change per 10 °C (10 K) rise	Q_{10}	
chemical shift	δ	
chemical terminology and symbols		see Refs 1, 2
chi-squared (statistics)	χ^2	with stated number of degrees of freedom
chorionic gonadotropin (gonadotrophin)	CG	see '-trophic/-trophin'
clearance	C	e.g. C_{PAH}, C_{urea}, C_{Cr}
clinical biochemical nomenclature		see Refs 13, 14
cobalamin derivatives		vitamin B_{12} *preferred* for consideration of biological activity
coefficient	coeff.	
coenzyme A	CoA	
coenzyme I		*use* NAD, etc.; see Refs 1, 2
coenzyme II		*use* NADP, etc.; see Refs 1,2
colony-stimulating factor	CSF	
granulocyte	G-CSF	
granulocyte–macrophage	GM-CSF	
macrophage	M-CSF	
complement components	e.g. C1q	
complement receptors	e.g. CR1	
complete blood count	CBC	full blood count (FBC) is *preferred* in UK/European usage
compliance (respiratory)	C	
compound	cpd	in titles of medicinal preparations, 'Co.' is conventionally used
compressibility (bulk)	κ	
computed tomography	CT	*not* CAT
concentrated	conc.	

concentration	concn	
amount of substance	c	of substance B, c_B
mass	ρ	of substance B, ρ_B
unspecified	C	
of given substance	[ ]	e.g. [H⁺], [urea], [HCO₃]

conductance:		
electrical	g	
thermal	G	

conductivity:		
electrical	σ	
thermal	κ	

confidence interval, 95%	95% CI
confidence limits, 95%	95% CL
constant	const
corrected	corr.

correlation coefficient:		
of hypothetical population	ρ	
of observed sample	r	

counts per minute	counts/min *or* cpm, *or* c.p.m.
covariance	Cov *or* cov
C-reactive protein	CRP
creatinine	Cr
creatinine clearance	C_{Cr}
critical	crit.
critical value	c *or* cr *or* crit
crystalline	cryst.
cubic	cu.
cubic centimetre	
curie	Ci
current density	J
cycles per second	c/s
cyclooxygenase	COX

Right-column notes:

- creatinine clearance — *preferred to* CrCl
- critical value — as subscript – in roman (upright) type
- cubic — *avoid* with units
- cubic centimetre — *avoid* cc; *use* cm³ *or* (except for results of high precision) mL (*or* ml)
- curie — *avoid*; *use* becquerel (1 Ci = 3.7 × 10¹⁰ Bq)
- cycles per second — *avoid*; *use* hertz (Hz)
- cyclooxygenase — e.g. COX-1

cysteine	Cys, C	
cytosine	C	
cytidine	C	deoxycytidine: dC
cytotoxic T lymphocyte	CTL	
dalton (atomic mass unit)	Da	see Table 1.5; *avoid* D (which is the abbreviation for the debye, a non-SI unit of dipole moment); may also be used for the mass of a complex entity (e.g. a ribosome)
date		3 October 1924 is unambiguous; if only digits are used, the ISO recommendation is 1924-10-03 *or* 19241003
day	d	*avoid* if an alternative meaning is 'day in contrast to night' (e.g. for excretion of urine); if necessary, *use* 24 h
dead-space volume	V_D	
decay/disintegration constant	λ	reciprocal of mean life
decibel	dB	
decimal point	·	on the line; the use of the comma as the decimal marker is widespread internationally – therefore the comma must *not* be used as a spacer for grouping figures in thousands in English texts (*avoid* e.g. 10,000); see Chapter 1
decomposition	decomp.	
degree Celsius	°C	*not* 'centigrade'; see Table 1.2
degree Fahrenheit	°F	also give Celsius or kelvin equivalent
degree Kelvin	°K	*avoid*; *use* kelvin (K) for both thermodynamic temperature and temperature interval
degrees of freedom (statistics)	df *or* d.f.	
denaturing gradient gel electrophoresis	DGGE	
density (mass)	ρ	
deoxyribonuclease	DNase	*avoid* DNAase and DNAse

deoxyribonucleic acid	DNA	
complementary	cDNA	
double-stranded	dsDNA	
mitochondrial	mtDNA	
ribosomal	rDNA	*avoid* rDNA for recombinant DNA
deoxyribose	dRib	
dextro-:		
configuration	D-	
optical rotation	(+)-	
dextrose		*avoid; use* glucose
diacylglycerol	DAG	
dialysate		*avoid; use* diffusate
diameter	D *or* d	
inside	ID *or* i.d.	
outside	OD *or* o.d.	
diffusing capacity of lung	D_L	
diffusion coefficient	D	
for lung	K	
digital subtraction angiography	DSA	
dimethylsulphoxide	DMSO	
dioptre	D	
prism	Δ	
direct current	DC *or* d.c.	
disease, nomenclature of		there is no universally used system, but see Refs 15, 16
disintegrations per minute	d/min *or* dpm *or* d.p.m.	
dissociation, degree of	α	
dissociation constant:		
negative logarithm of	pK	
acidic	K_a	
apparent	K_a'	
basic	K_b	
substrate–enzyme	K_s	
dopamine receptors	D_1, etc.	
drug concentration (e.g. in plasma)		*preferably use* substance (not mass) concentration (e.g. mmol/L)
drug dose frequency		*preferably use* e.g. 'three times daily' *or* '8-hourly' rather than Latin terms such as 'ter in die (t.i.d.)'

drug names		generic (non-proprietary) names should always be used, with the proprietary name (with first letter capitalized) following in parentheses if necessary
international		for International Nonproprietary Names (INNs), see Refs 17, 18
UK		for British Approved Names (BANs), see Refs 18–20
US		for United States Adopted Names (USANs), see Ref 18
dry ice		*use* 'solid CO_2'
dual-energy X-ray absorptiometry	DXA	*preferred to* DEXA
echo time (magnetic resonance imaging)	TE	TE1, etc. for multiple echoes
effective dose, median	ED_{50}	
elastance	E	
electric current	I	
electrocardiogram	ECG	some American authors use EKG
electroencephalogram	EEG	
electromotive force (emf, e.m.f.)	E *or* $\mathscr{E}$	
electromyogram	EMG	
electron microscopy	EM	
scanning	SEM	
transmission	TEM	
electron paramagnetic resonance	EPR	
electron spin resonance	ESR	
energy	E	
heat; radiant	Q	
kinetic (KE, k.e.)	E_k	often denoted by T in physics
potential (PE, p.e.)	E_p	often denoted by V in physics
enzyme-linked immunosorbent assay	ELISA	
enzyme-multiplied immunoassay test	EMIT	
enzyme terminology		see Refs 21–23

enzyme unit (international)	U	as micromoles of substrate transformed or product formed per minute under specified conditions, which must be defined
enzymatic catalytic activity		SI unit, katal: as moles (of substrate or product change) per second, under defined conditions
equilibrium constant	K	
equivalent (general use)	equiv.	
equivalent (unit of substance)	Eq	*avoid*; *use* mole
epidermal growth factor	EGF	
erythrocyte sedimentation rate	ESR	
erythropoietin	EPO	
estrogen receptor	ER	*use* ER also when using 'oestrogen' spelling
ethanol		*not* ethyl alcohol
ethylenediamine tetraacetic acid	EDTA	
exchangeable	a (subscript)	e.g. Na_a
experiment/al	expt/l	
expired minute ventilation	$\dot{V}_E$	
exponential (of x)	$\exp(x)$ *or* e^x	*use* $\exp(x)$ if x is itself a complicated expression (especially if it contains subscripts and superscripts)
extinction	E	*use* absorbance
extinction coefficient, molar	ε	
extracellular fluid	ECF	
factor (coagulation)	e.g. FV	activated form indicated by suffix a: e.g. FVa
Faraday constant	F	
fast Fourier transform	FFT	

fatty acids:
   free
   non-esterified
	
	FFA
	NEFA	

fibroblast growth factor
   acidic
   basic
	FGF
	aFGF
	bFGF	

23

filtered load of x	F_x	
flow rate: 　average 　instantaneous	$\dot{V}$ $\dot{v}$	for volume
fluid ounce	fl oz	*avoid*; *use* SI equivalent: 1 fl oz (UK) $\approx$28 mL; 1 fl oz (US) $\approx$30 mL
fluorescein isothiocyanate	FITC	
fluorescence in situ hybridization	FISH	
flux	J	
folic acid and derivatives		folacin *preferred* as generic descriptor for biological activities
follicle-stimulating hormone	FSH	
foot	ft	*avoid*; *use* SI equivalent (1 ft $\approx$0.3 m)
force	F	
forced expiratory volume	FEV	e.g. $FEV_{0.5}$, in 0.5 s
fractional concentration in dry gas	F	
fractional disappearance rate	k	
freezing point	f.p.	*preferred to* fp
frequency 　circular (pulsatance) 　of respiration	f *or* v ω f_R	ω is also used for angular velocity
friction, coefficient of	μ	
fructose	Fru	
fucose	Fuc	
full blood count	FBC	*preferred to* complete blood count (CBC) in UK/European usage
galactose	Gal	
gallon		*avoid*; *use* SI equivalent: 1 gallon (UK) $\approx$4.5 L; 1 gallon (US) $\approx$3.8 L
gamma (magnetic flux density)	γ	*avoid*; *use* nanotesla (nT)
gamma (mass)	γ	*avoid*; *use* microgram (μg)

γ-aminobutyric acid	GABA	
γ-aminobutyric acid receptors	GABA$_A$, etc.	
gas constant, per mole	R	
gas–liquid chromatography	GLC	
gas transfer factor	T	

gene nomenclature:
  human
  mouse and rat
		see Refs 24, 25
		see Ref 26

generations (for pedigrees, etc.)		*use* roman numerals: I, II, … (but F_1, F_2, …); for individual subjects in each generation, *use* Arabic numerals: 1, 2, …
genus new	gen. gen.nov.	
Gibbs free energy	G	
glomerular filtration rate	GFR	
glucose	Glc	*avoid* Glu (glutamic acid); *preferred to* G, which may be used for brevity when no confusion is possible with guanosine or glycine
glutamic acid	Glu, E	
glutamine	Gln, Q	
glycine	Gly, G	
gram	g	*not* gm; 'gram' is now the accepted UK spelling for the unit, and is also used in compound words; 'gramme' is the Continental spelling
gram-ion		*avoid*: *use* mole
gram-molecule		*avoid*; *use* mole
green fluorescent protein	GFP	
growth hormone	GH	*preferred to* somatotrophin, STH
guanine	G	
guanosine	G	deoxyguanosine: dG

guanosine 5′-monophosphate	GMP	
5′-diphosphate	GDP	
5′-triphosphate	GTP	
cyclic 3′:5′-monophosphate	cGMP	
gyromagnetic ratio	γ	
haematocrit	Hct	packed cell volume (PCV) is *preferred*
haematological terminology		see Ref 27
haematoxylin and eosin	H&E *or* HE	
haemoglobin	Hb	
oxyhaemoglobin	HbO_2	
carboxyhaemoglobin	HbCO	
methaemoglobin	Hi	
half-body radiation	HBR	
half disappearance time	h.d.t.	
half-life:		
nuclear physics	$T_{\frac{1}{2}}$	
biological	$t_{\frac{1}{2}}$	
half-value layer	HVL	
half-value thickness	HVT	
hazard ratio	HR	
heat	Q	
heat capacity	C	
height	$H \ or \ h$	
helix–loop–helix	HLH	
high frequency	HF *or* h.f.	
high-performance (-pressure) liquid chromatography	HPLC	
histamine receptors	H_1, etc.	
histidine	His, H	
hormone terminology		see Ref 19
(hormone)-releasing hormone	( )RH	e.g. LHRH, GnRH; -relin is used in pharmacy
(hormone)-release inhibiting factor	( )RIF	-statin (as suffix)

human (for hormones)	h	e.g. hPL (human placental lactogen)
human leucocyte antigen	HLA	e.g. HLA-B27; for detailed nomenclature, see Ref 28
human serum albumin	HSA	
humidity:		
absolute (physiology)	γ	
relative	ϕ	
hydrogen ion activity	a_H	
negative logarithm (base 10) of numerical value (hydrogen ion exponent)	pH	plural: 'pH values' (similarly for pNa, etc.)
3-hydroxy-3-methylglutaryl coenzyme A	HMG-CoA	
immunoglobulins	IgA, IgD, IgE, IgG, IgM	subclasses: IgA1, IgA2; IgG1, …, IgG4
immunoradiometric assay	IRMA	
impedance	Z	
inch	in	*avoid*; *use* SI equivalent (1 in = 25.4 mm); do not abbreviate if confusion possible with preposition 'in'
increment (finite)	Δ	
infective dose, for 50%	ID_{50}	
infrared	IR	
inhibitor/inhibition constant	K_i	
inhibitory concentration/dose giving 50% maximal	IC_{50}/ID_{50}	
inorganic phosphate	P_i	
inositol trisphosphate	IP_3	
insoluble	insol.	
insulin-like growth factor	IGF	e.g. IGF-1
intelligence quotient	IQ	
intercellular adhesion molecule	ICAM	
interferon	IFN	e.g. IFN-α
interleukin	IL	e.g. IL-1

international unit	IU *or* iu	*preferably* also give SI equivalent in clinical writing; *always* do so in scientific writing
intra-arterial	IA *or* i.a.	
intracellular fluid	ICF	
intramuscular	IM *or* i.m.	
intraperitoneal	IP *or* i.p.	
intravenous	IV *or* i.v.	
inversion time (magnetic resonance imaging)	TI	
ionic charge		e.g. Ca^{2+} *not* Ca^{++}
ionic strength	I	
isoelectric point	pI	
isoenzyme		*preferred to* isozyme; the enzyme that runs fastest towards the anode on electrophoresis is numbered isoenzyme-1
isoleucine	Ile, I	
isotonic		give composition
isotope (atomic mass) labelling		left superscript, e.g. iodine-131 = ^{131}I; metastable nuclear isomers are indicated by 'm', e.g. technetium-99m = ^{99m}Tc *or* $^{99}Tc^{m}$
isotopically labelled compounds		when exact chemical nature of substitution is uncertain or name of substances labelled is descriptive rather than chemical, *use* e.g. ^{131}I-labelled albumin (*preferred to* ^{131}I-albumin), ^{51}Cr-labelled erythrocytes
isotopically substituted compounds		indicate isotope in formula, e.g. $^{3}H_2O$, $Na^{99m}TcO_4$; or give substituting atom in square brackets before name of compound, e.g. $[^{18}F]$2-fluoro-2-deoxy-D-glucose, $[^{14}C]$urea see Refs 1, 2, 29

kilocalorie	kcal	may be used only in nutrition – otherwise *avoid*; *use* kilojoule (1 kcal = 4.184 kJ); do *not* use Calorie (Cal) as a synonym for kilocalorie
kilovoltage:		
peak	kV_p	
generated at constant potential	kV_{cp}	
kilowatt hour	kW h	*preferably use* joule (1 kW h = 3.6 MJ); the kW h is used for energy consumption of equipment
Krebs cycle		*use* tricarboxylic acid cycle *or* citric acid cycle
lactate dehydrogenase	LDH *or* LD	
laevo-:		
configuration	L-	
optical rotation	(–)-	
lambda (volume)	λ	*avoid*; *use* microlitre (μL, μl) or cubic millimetre (mm^3)
laevulose		*avoid*; *use* fructose
length	*L or l*	
lethal dose, median	LD_{50}	
leucine	Leu, L	
linear energy transfer (LET)	*L*	
lipoprotein:		
high-density	HDL	
low-density	LDL	
very low-density	VLDL	
litre	L *or* l	see Table 1.4
locus control region	LCR	
logarithm:		
any base	log	
base 2	log_2	
base 10	log_{10} *or* lg	
base e (natural)	log_e *or* ln	
long-term potentiation	LTP	
long terminal repeat	LTR	
loss of heterozygosity	LOH	

loudness level	L_N	
low frequency	LF *or* l.f.	
luminous flux	Φ	
luminous intensity	I *or* I_v	
luteinizing hormone	LH	
luteotropin (luteotrophin)		*avoid; use* prolactin
lysine	Lys, K	
magnetic field gradients (magnetic resonance imaging)	G_x, G_y, G_z	
magnetic field strength	H	see Refs 30, 31 for usage of H and B in magnetic resonance imaging
magnetic flux density (magnetic induction)	B	
magnetic resonance	MR	
magnetic resonance angiography	MRA	
magnetic resonance imaging functional	MRI fMRI	for terminology, see Refs 30, 31
magnetic resonance spectroscopy	MRS	
magnetization (magnetic resonance imaging): longitudinal transverse	M_z M_{xy}	
major histocompatibility complex	MHC	
mannose	Man	
mass	M *or* m	
mass flow rate	q_m	
mass fraction (of compound B)	w_B	
maximal tubular (reabsorption, etc.)	Tm	e.g. Tm_{PAH}
maximum	max.	
mean corpuscular haemoglobin	MCH	
mean corpuscular haemoglobin concentration	MCHC	

mean corpuscular volume	MCV	
mean life (atomic physics)	τ	
mean value	$^{-}$	e.g. mean value of x: $\bar{x}$

mean value:
    of hypothetical population
    of observed sample
	μ
	m	

melanocyte-stimulating hormone	MSH	
melting point	m.p.	*preferred to* mp
menaquinone and derivatives		vitamin K *preferred* as generic descriptor for biological activities
meta-	*m-*	
metabolic quotient	Q	*avoid* Q_x, *etc.; preferably use* e.g. mmol s^{-1} mg^{-1}, etc.
methanol		*not* methyl alcohol
methionine	Met, M	
mho	℧	*avoid; use* siemens (S)
Michaelis constant	K_m	
micron	μ	*avoid; use* micrometre (μm)
mile		*avoid; use* SI equivalent: 1 statute mile $\approx$1.61 km; 1 nautical mile $\approx$1.85 km *do not* abbreviate
miles per hour	mph	*avoid; use* SI equivalent (1 mph $\approx$1.61 km/h)
milliequivalent	mEq	*avoid; use* millimole (mmol)
millilitre	mL *or* ml	see Table 1.4
millimetre of mercury	mmHg	use only when conventional, and measurement has been made with a mercury (column) manometer, e.g. for blood pressure; note that the mmHg is a legal unit for measurement of blood pressure in some countries; *preferably* also give SI equivalent (1 mmHg = 133.322 Pa)
millimole	mmol	*not* mM or mM (which mean mmol/L)
milliosmole	mosmol	millimole (mmol) is *preferred*

minimal inhibitory concentration/dose	MIC/MID	
minimum	min.	
mitogen-activated protein kinase kinase kinase kinase kinase kinase	MAPK MAP2K *or* MAPKK MAP3K *or* MAPKKK	
mobility (electrophoresis)	*m*	
molal		*avoid*; *use* mol/kg
molality of solute substance B	*m* m_B	
molar (concentration)	M	*preferably use* mol/L; 'molar' strictly means 'divided by amount of substance', and *preferably* should not be used for concentration, but rather to mean 'per mole' (as in 'molar conductivity')
molar mass	*M*	
mole (unit of amount of substance)	mol	*not* M or M (which mean mol/L); replaces gram-molecule, gram-ion, gram-formula, gram-atom, etc.
molecular biology nomenclature		see Refs 1, 2
molecular mass		the appropriate unit is the dalton (Da); see Table 1.5
molecular weight	MW	alternative term for 'relative molecular mass (M_r)', the ratio of the molecular mass to the mass of a ^{12}C atom; it is a numerical ratio and does *not* have the unit 'dalton'
moment of inertia	*I*	
morgan	M	unit of genetic distance: 1 cM = 1% of crossovers
muscarinic receptors	M_1, etc.	
neural cell adhesion molecule	NCAM *or* N-CAM	
neuraminic acid	Neu	
nicotinic acid and derivatives		niacin *preferred* as generic descriptor for biological activity

N-methyl-D-aspartate	NMDA	
normal (concentration)	N	*avoid*; give concentration in mol/L
normal range		*avoid*; *use* reference range *or* reference interval
normal saline		*avoid*; *use* 0.9% saline
normal temperature and pressure		*avoid*; *use* standard temperature and pressure
northern blot, northwestern blot		'n' is *not* capitalized (techniques are named in analogy to Southern blot)
not significant	NS	
nuclear factor κB	NFκB *or* NF-κB	
nuclear magnetic resonance	NMR	
nucleosides and nucleotides		see Refs 1, 2
number density (of molecules or particles)	*n*	
number of haploid chromosomes	n	
number of molecules (or other elementary entities)	*N*	
number of moles (amount of substance)	*n*	
number of observations (statistics)	*n*	
numbers, large and small – expression of		*either* with powers of ten *or* grouped in threes without commas, e.g. one and a half million = 1.5×10^6 *or* 1 500 000; see also Chapter 1. For high and low values of units, *use* appropriate prefixes (see Table 1.3), chosen so that the resulting numerical value is between 0.1 and 1000, e.g. 1.5×10^6 volts = 1.5 MV
numerical aperture	NA *or* n.a.	
observed	obs.	
odds ratio	OR	
oestrogen receptor	ER	*not* OR

one-dimensional	1D	*preferred to* 1-D, 1d, 1-d
optical density	D	only for non-monochromatic light or for suspensions; otherwise *use* absorbance
optical rotation	α	
optimum	opt.	
ortho-	*o-*	
osmole	osmol	mole is *preferred*
osmotic pressure	Π	
ounce	oz	*avoid*; *use* SI equivalent (1 oz $\approx$28 g)
oxygen consumption	Q_{O_2}	measured as μL per mg dry mass per hour
	n_{O_2}	as mol s^{-1}
packed cell volume	PCV	*preferred to* haematocrit (Hct)
para-	*p-*	
parathyroid hormone	PTH	
partial pressure	P	e.g. P_{CO_2} and Pa_{CO_2} (arterial); *preferred to* p, to avoid confusion with p as in pH; note that p is customary in physical sciences
partial specific volume	v	
partial thromboplastin time	PTT	*preferably use* activated partial thromboplastin time (APTT *or* aPTT)
parts per million	ppm *or* p.p.m. *or* parts/10^6	*preferably use* appropriate SI concentration
pathology (especially histopathology) terminology		see Ref 16
peak expiratory flow rate	PEFR	
per cent *or* percent	%	*or* in full; *do not use* for /100 mL or /100 g; *avoid* for concentrations of solutions
per thousand		*avoid* ‰; *preferably* write in full
period (time, of a periodically varying quantity)	T	
periodic acid–Schiff reagent	PAS	

34

permeability:		
physiology	P	
magnetic	μ	
petroleum ether		*avoid*; *use* light petroleum (give b.p. range)
pharmacokinetics terminology and symbols		see Ref 32
phenylalanine	Phe, F	
phonocardiogram	PCG	
phosphatidylinositol 3′-kinase	PI3K *or* PI3-K	
physics terminology and symbols		see Ref 29
pint		*avoid*; *use* SI equivalent: 1 pint (UK) ≈568 mL 1 pint (US) ≈473 mL
plasma (e.g. laboratory reporting)	P	
plasma concentration	P *or* C_p	usually with subscript, e.g. P_{urea} *or* $C_{p,urea}$
plasminogen activator	PA	
tissue-type	tPA *or* t-PA	
urokinase-type	uPA *or* u-PA	
plasminogen activator inhibitor	PAI	
platelet-derived growth factor	PDGF	
polymerase chain reaction	PCR	
reverse transcriptase	RT–PCR	
positron emission tomography	PET	
posterior	post.	
post meridiem	p.m.	24-hour clock *preferred*
potential difference	V	
pound	lb	*avoid*; *use* SI equivalent (1 lb ≈0.45 kg)
preparation	prep.	
probability, in statistical hypothesis testing	P *or* p	conventional notation is *, $p < 0.05$; **, $p < 0.01$; ***, $p < 0.001$
progesterone receptor	PgR *or* PR	
prolactin	PRL	
proline	Pro, P	

prostacyclin (i.e. 'prostaglandin I_2')	PGI_2	
prostaglandin	PG	e.g. $PGF_{2\alpha}$
prostate-specific antigen	PSA	
protein kinase A, B, C	PKA, PKB, PKC	PKB is also known as Akt
prothrombin time	PT	
pulsed-field gel electrophoresis	PFGE	
pyridoxine/pyridoxal		vitamin B_6 *preferred* for consideration of biological activity
radian	rad	see also Table 1.2, footnote *d*
radiant flux	Φ	
radiant intensity	I *or* I_e	
radiation absorbed dose	rad *or* rd	*avoid*; *use* gray (1 rad = 0.01 Gy)
radiation dose equivalent	rem	'radiation equivalent man' (for protection purposes): *avoid*; *use* sievert (1 rem = 0.01 Sv)
radioimmunoassay	RIA	
radius	R *or* r	
randomly labelled	r.l.	
rate constant	k	
rate of reaction	v	
reaction time (neurophysiology)	RT	
receptor	R *or* -R	as suffix, e.g. PDGFR *or* PDGF-R (platelet-derived growth factor receptor)
recrystallized	recryst.	
red blood cell	RBC	*avoid* corpuscle; erythrocyte is *preferred*
redox potential	E'_o	
refractive index	n	
relative atomic mass	A_r	a numerical ratio; it does *not* have the unit 'dalton'

relative band speed (chromatography):		
to front	R_F	
to reference compound X	R_X	
relative biological effectiveness	RBE	
relative density	d	reference conditions must be clear
relative humidity	r.h.	
relative mobility (electrophoresis)	M, M_X	
relative molecular mass	M_r	'molecular weight'; a numerical ratio; it does *not* have the unit 'dalton'
relative retention time (gas chromatography)	t_r	
relative risk	RR	
relaxation times (magnetic resonance imaging):		
longitudinal (spin–lattice)	T_1 *or* T1	
transverse (spin–spin)	T_2 *or* T2	
effective transverse	T_2^* *or* T2*	
remainder	rem.	
renal plasma flow	RPF	
repetition time (magnetic resonance imaging)	TR	
resistance, electrical or rheological	R	
respiratory exchange ratio	R	
respiratory frequency	f_R	
respiratory physiology (terminology and symbols)		see Ref 33
respiratory quotient	RQ	
restriction fragment length polymorphism	RFLP	
retinol and derivatives		vitamin A *preferred* as generic descriptor for consideration of biological activity
revolutions per minute	rpm *or* r.p.m. *or* rev min^{-1} *or* rev/min	*use g* for centrifugal conditions

riboflavin		*use* also for consideration of biological activity
ribonucleic acid	RNA	
double-stranded	dsRNA	
messenger	mRNA	
mitochondrial	mtRNA	
nuclear	nRNA	
ribosomal	rRNA	
single-stranded	ssRNA	
small nuclear	snRNA	
small nucleolar	snoRNA	
transfer	tRNA	
ribose	Rib	
röntgen	R	*avoid*; *use* SI units ($1\ R = 2.58 \times 10^{-4}$ C/kg)
root mean square	RMS *or* rms *or* r.m.s.	
saline		give composition; *avoid* 'normal' (*use* '0.9%'); 'isotonic' or 'isoosmotic' is *preferred* (when appropriate) to 'physiological'
saturated	sat.	
saturation	S	e.g. Sao_2 (arterial oxygen saturation)
sedimentation coefficient (ultracentrifugation)	s	
serine	Ser, S	
serotonin (5-hydroxytryptamine)	5-HT	
serotonin receptors	5-HT_1, etc.	
serum (e.g. laboratory reporting)	S	
single nucleotide polymorphism	SNP	
single photon emission computed tomography	SPECT	
single-strand conformational polymorphism	SSCP	
sodium dodecyl sulphate polyacrylamide gel electrophoresis	SDS SDS–PAGE	

solidus	/	for the use of the solidus in unit abbreviations, see Chapter 1
soluble	sol.	
solution	soln	
solvent systems		e.g. ethanol/water (4:1, v/v); by vol is *preferred* if there are more than two components
sound intensity	*J*	
Southern blot		capital 'S' (technique is named after its inventor)
southwestern blot		's' is *not* capitalized (technique is named in analogy to Southern blot)
species	sp.	
plural	spp.	
new	sp.nov.	
specific	sp.	in physics means 'divided by mass'
specific activity	sp.act.	
specific gravity	sp.gr.	relative density is *preferred*
specific heat (capacity)	*c*	
spinal segments	C1, … T1, … L1, … S1, … Co1, …	
square(d)	sq.	*avoid* with units
standard deviation:		
of hypothetical population	σ	
of observed sample	SD *or s*	
standard error (of estimate of mean value)	SEM	*preferred to* s.e.mean; *not* ±
standard temperature and pressure	STPD	(dry)
standard wire gauge	SWG *or* s.w.g.	give dimensions in SI units
steradian	sr	*not* 'srad'; see also Table 1.2, footnote *d*
stone		*avoid*; *use* SI equivalent (1 stone ≈6.35 kg)
strain (taxonomy)	str.	

strain:		
linear	ε	
shear	γ	
volume	θ	
stress:		
normal	σ	
shear	τ	
Student's t (statistics)	t	with stated number of degrees of freedom
subcutaneous	SC *or* s.c.	
sugars and derivatives		see Refs 1, 2
sum	Σ	e.g. $\sum_i x_i$
sum, statistical:		
of hypothetical population	Σ	
of observed sample	$s\ or\ \Sigma$	
surface tension	σ	
Svedberg flotation unit	S_f	
Svedberg unit	S	0.1 ps
T-cell receptor	TCR	
technical error of a measurement (statistics)	t.e.	
teeth, symbols for		name in full (e.g. right upper canine); but see Ref 34
temperature:		
thermodynamic	T	
other (Celsius customary)	t	where t is required for time, θ may be used for temperature
tension, of gases in liquids (physiology)		*use* partial pressure, e.g. P_{CO_2}, P_{O_2}
thermal conductivity	κ	
thermal diffusivity	α	
thermal resistance	R	
thiamin		also *preferred to* vitamin B_1 for consideration of biological activity
thin-layer chromatography	TLC	

three-dimensional	3D	*preferred to* 3-D, 3d, 3-d
threonine	Thr, T	
thrombin time	TT	also known as thrombin clotting time: TCT
thromboxane	Tx	e.g. TxA_2
thymine	T	
thymidine	dT	thymidine is the *deoxy*ribonucleoside; the abbreviation T represents ribosyl-thymine (the ribonucleoside)
thyroid-stimulating hormone	TSH	*or* thyrotropin (thyrotrophin); see '-trophic/-trophin'
thyroxine	T_4	
tidal volume	V_T	
time	t	
time of day		e.g. 18:30, *or* 1830 if unambiguous; *not* 18.30 h
time constant (of an changing quantity)	τ	
time, periodic	T	
time, rate of change with	$\cdot$	e.g. $\dot{V}$ (rate of change of gas volume, change in gas volume per unit time)
tissue factor	TF	
tocopherol		vitamin E *preferred* for consideration of biological activity
torr	Torr	*avoid*; *use* SI units (1 Torr $\approx$ 1 mmHg = 133.322 Pa)
total iron-binding capacity	TIBC	
transcutaneous	Tc	
transfer factor	T	
transforming growth factor	TGF	e.g. TGF-β
transmittance	T	
triiodothyronine reverse	T_3 rT_3	
-trophic/-trophin (in hormone names)		the alternative endings -tropic/-tropin are *preferred* for use internationally for all such hormones
tryptophan	Trp, W	

tubular maximal reabsorptive capacity, for x	Tm_x	
tumour necrosis factor	TNF	e.g. TNF-α
two-dimensional	2D	*preferred to* 2-D, 2d, 2-d
tyrosine	Tyr, Y	
ultraviolet	UV	
uncorrected	uncorr.	
unit	u	*preferred to* U, which should be reserved for 'enzyme unit'; to be used, when unavoidable, for arbitrary units, which must be defined; in atomic physics, the symbol u means 'unified atomic mass unit'
untranslated region	UTR	
uracil	U	
urea and electrolytes	U&E	
uridine	U	deoxyuridine: dU
urinary concentration	U *or* C_u	usually with subscript, e.g. U_{urea} *or* $C_{u, urea}$
urine (e.g. laboratory reporting)	U	
vacuum	vac.	
valency		e.g. divalent (ferrous) iron: as ionic charge: Fe^{2+} as oxidation number: iron(II), Fe^{II}
valine		Val, V
vanillylmandelic acid	VMA	*or* 4-hydroxy-3-methoxymandelic acid (HMMA)
vapour density	v.d.	
vapour pressure	v.p.	
variance ratio (statistics)	F	with stated number of degrees of freedom
variety (biology)	var.	
vascular cell adhesion molecule	VCAM *or* V-CAM	
vasoactive intestinal peptide	VIP	

vascular endothelial growth factor	VEGF	
velocity:		
angular	ω	
linear	υ	
venous	v	
ventilation (volume per minute)	$\dot{V}$	e.g. $\dot{V}\text{CO}_2$
ventilation/perfusion	$\dot{V}/\dot{Q}$	
viral nomenclature		see Refs 35, 36
viscosity:		
dynamic	η	
kinematic	ν	
vitamins		see under individual chemical names
void volume	V_o	
volume	V	
liquid phase (physiology)	Q	e.g. Q_c (capillary blood flow rate)
volume per volume	v/v	only for two components; otherwise *use* 'by vol.'; *preferably* specify units
von Willebrand factor	vWF	*preferred to* VWF
wavelength	λ	
weight	wt	often used conventionally, but wrongly, for mass: weight involves gravitational attraction
weight by volume	w/v	mass/vol. is correct, or *use* mass concentration; *preferably* specify units
western blot		'w' is *not* capitalized (technique is named in analogy to Southern blot)
white blood cell	WBC	*avoid* corpuscle; leucocyte is *preferred* (the alternative spelling leukocyte is often used internationally)
work	W	
xylose	Xyl	
yard	yd	*avoid*; *use* SI equivalent (1 yd ≈0.91 m)

year	a	this is the international symbol, although yr is conventional in English-language publications; *preferably* do not abbreviate
Young's modulus (elasticity)	*E*	
zoological and veterinary nomenclature		see Refs 4–6

References

1. Instructions to Authors for *Biochemical Journal* available at www.biochemj. org/bj/bji2a.htm.
2. Liebecq C, ed. *Compendium of Biochemical Nomenclature and Related Documents,* 2nd edn. London: Portland Press, 1992.
3. International Committee of Anatomical Terminology. *Terminologica Anatomica.* Stuttgart: Thieme, 1998.
4. Festing MFW. *International Index of Laboratory Animals,* 6th edn. Leicester, UK: MFW Festing, 1993.
5. International Commission on Zoological Nomenclature. *International Code of Zoological Nomenclature,* 4th edn. London: International Trust for Zoological Nomenclature/Natural History Museum, 1999. Available at www.iczn.org/iczn/ index.jsp.
6. International Committee on Veterinary Gross Anatomical Nomenclature. *Nomina Anatomica Veterinaria,* 5th edn. Hannover, Columbia, Gent, Sapporo: ICVGAN, 2005. Available at www.wava-amav.org/nav.htm.
7. Skerman VBD, McGowan V, Sneath PHA, eds. *Approved List of Bacterial Names.* Washington, DC: American Society for Microbiology, 1989. Available at www.ncbi.nlm.nih.gov/sites/entrez?db=books.
8. Garrity GM et al, eds. *Bergey's Manual of Systemic Bacteriology,* 2nd edn, Vols 1–. New York: Springer-Verlag, 2001–.
9. International Society of Blood Transfusion Committee on Terminology for Red Cell Surface Antigens. ISBT Terminology and Workshops. Available at www.blood.co.uk/ibgrl.
10. Daniels GL, Fletcher A, Garraty G, et al. Blood group terminology 2004: from the International Society of Blood Transfusion Committee on Terminology for Red Cell Surface Antigens. *Vox Sang* 2004; **87**: 304–16.
11. Klein HG, Anstee DJ. *Mollison's Blood Transfusion in Clinical Medicine,* 11th edn. Oxford: Blackwell, 2005.
12. McNeill J, Barrie FR, Burdet HM, et al, eds *International Code of Botanical Nomenclature (Vienna Code).* International Association for Plant Taxonomy, Regnum Vegetabile 246. Ruggell: Gantner Verlag, 2006. Available at ibot.sav.sk/icbn/main.htm.
13. Rigg JC, Brown SS, Dybkaer R, Oleson H *Compendium of Terminology and Nomenclature of Properties in Clinical Laboratory Sciences – The Silver Book.* Commission on Quantities and Units in Clinical Chemistry of the International Union of

Pure and Applied Chemistry and the International Federation of Clinical Chemistry. Oxford: Blackwell Science, 1995.

14. Lehman HP, Fuentes-Arderiu X, Bertello LF. Glossary of terms in quantities and units in clinical chemistry (IUPAC–IFCC recommendations 1996). *Pure Appl Chem* 1996; **68**: 957–1000.

15. World Health Organization. *International Statistical Classification of Diseases and Health Related Problems, 10th Revision (ICD-10),* 2nd edn. Geneva: WHO, 2005. Available at www.who.int/classifications/icd/en.

16. Systematized Nomenclature of Medicine Clinical Terms (SNOMED CT). International Health Terminology Standards Development Organisation (IHTSDO). www.ihtsdo.org.

17. List of Recommended and Approved INNs. World Health Organization Drug Information. Available at www.who.int/druginformation/general/innlists.shtml.

18. *USP Pharmacopeia Dictionary of USAN and International Drug Names.* Rockville, MD: US Pharmacopeia, published yearly.

19. British Pharmacopoeia Commission. *British Approved Names 2007.* London: TSO (The Stationery Office), 2007.

20. *British National Formulary.* London: British Medical Association/Royal Pharmaceutical Society of Great Britain, published twice yearly. Available at www.bnf.org/bnf.

21. *Enzyme Nomenclature. Recommendations of the Nomenclature Committee of the International Union of Biochemistry and Molecular Biology.* London: Academic Press, 1992 and Supplements 1–5 in *Eur J Biochem* (1993–99). The updated web version is available at www.chem.qmul.ac.uk/iubmb/enzyme.

22. ENZYME: Enzyme Nomenclature Database. Available at www.expasy.ch/enzyme.

23. Baron DN, Moss DW, Walker PG, Wilkinson JH. Revised list of abbreviations for names of enzymes of diagnostic importance. *J Clin Pathol* 1975; **28**: 592–3.

24. HUGO Gene Nomenclature Committee (HGNC). Available at www.genenames.org/index.html.

25. Wain HM, Bruford EA, Lovering RC, Lush MJ, Wright MW, Povey S. Guidelines for human gene nomenclature. *Genomics* 2002; **79**: 464–70.

26. Mouse Genomic Nomenclature Committee (MGNC). Available at www.informatics.jax.org/mgihome/nomen.

27. Lewis SM, Bain BJ, Bates I. *Dacie and Lewis Practical Haematology,* 10th edn. Edinburgh: Churchill Livingstone, 2006.

28. Marsh SGE, Bodmer JG, Albert ED, et al. Nomenclature for factors of the HLA system, 2000. *Tissue Antigens* 2001; **57**: 236–83.

29. International Union of Pure and Applied Physics. *Symbols, Units, Nomenclature and Fundamental Constants in Physics (1987 Revision).* Document IUPAP-25. *Physica A* 1987; **146**: 1–68.

30. Instructions or Authors for *Magnetic Resonance in Medicine* and for *Journal of Magnetic Resonance Imaging.* Available at www.ismrm.org/journals.htm.

31. American College of Radiology. *ACR Glossary of MR Terms,* 4th edn. Reston, VA: ACR, 1995. See also www.acr.org (under 'Quality & Patient Safety').

32. Rowland M, Tucker G. Symbols in pharmacokinetics. *Br J Clin Pharmacol* 1982; **14**: 7–13.

33. Cotes JE, Chinn D, Miller MR. *Lung Function,* 6th edn. Oxford: Blackwell Scientific, 2006.

34. Sandham JA. The FDI two-digit system of designating teeth. *Int Dent J* 1983; **33**: 390–2.

35. Fauquet CM, Mayo MA, Maniloff J, Desselberger, U, Ball LA, eds. *Virus Taxonomy: Eighth Report of the International Committee on Taxonomy of Viruses.* San Diego: Elsevier Academic Press, 2005.
36. *Archives of Virology* Instructions to Authors. Available at www.springer.com/west/home/biomed?SGWID=4-124-70-1096244-D.

Note: Many of these references are periodically updated, and users should always consult the latest version.

Guides to nomenclature in many other special fields can be found in the following references:

- Lentner C, ed. *Geigy Scientific Tables*, 8th edn, Vols 1–6. Basle: Ciba-Geigy, 1981–92.
- Council of Science Editors. *Scientific Style and Format: The CSE Manual for Authors, Editors, and Publishers*, 7th edn. Reston, VA: CSE, 2006.
- Kotyk A. *Quantities, Symbols, Units, and Abbreviations in the Life Sciences – A Guide for Authors and Editors.* Totowa, NJ: Humana Press, 1999. This book does not always agree with our recommendations (e.g. with its long lists of abbreviations for names of diseases and syndromes), but is nevertheless useful.
- Iverson C, Christiansen S, Flanagin A et al. *AMA Manual of Style: A Guide for Authors and Editors*, 10th edn. New York: Oxford University Press, 2007.

3 | Layout of references

In this chapter, guidance is given on the organization and layout of references in journals, theses, and books.

It should always be remembered that a *reference* should be something to which the reader can *refer*, for checking or elucidation, preferably without undue difficulty. Therefore 'personal communication' should not be used in journal articles or in books, unless this is absolutely unavoidable, and should *never* be used in theses.

Journals

Submission to a journal is nowadays usually by electronic means, i.e. website or (for a few journals) email, rather than on paper as traditionally, although a number of journals will accept disk or (occasionally) paper as an alternative. The individual journal's most recent Instructions to Authors must be consulted, especially regarding illustrations and the system for references. Most major general journals in the biomedical sciences now use the Vancouver (citation-sequence) system, with minor variations in style, for citation of references in the text and for listing at the end of the contribution. The formerly almost universal and popular Harvard (name-and-year) system, which needs much more space in the text, is now primarily used for specialist journals.

Vancouver system

This is called after a conference of editors of major English-language general medical journals that was held in Vancouver in 1978. The system that they agreed upon has since been modified in minor ways, and journals still use a variety of different formats. Prospective authors should check before submitting to a particular journal (although changes in minor details will be made by the journal once an article has been accepted, it is better to avoid the need for this).

Only a brief outline of this preferred reference system will be given here; a valuable fuller description can be found in 'Uniform Requirements for Manuscripts Submitted to Biomedical Journals', produced by the International Committee of Medical Journal Editors and available at www.icmje.org (and, in a slightly different version, at thelancet.com/authors/uniform). This includes guidelines on referencing material other than articles and books in standard medical and scientific literature, such as websites, conference proceedings, newspaper articles, and law cases. It should be noted that there are innumerable minor variations between journals with regard to the detailed format of entries in reference lists, especially in the use of italic versus upright type for journal/book titles and bold versus normal type for volume numbers, and in punctuation within the entry. The following are therefore illustrative examples of an acceptable reference format.

Text citations

References are numbered in the order of their appearance in the text. They are usually indicated by superscript numbers, separated by commas (or, for a consecutive series, the first and last numbers, separated by a dash); on-line numbers in parentheses or square brackets are sometimes used. Papers by the authors 'in preparation' may be quoted as such in the text, but should not be listed.

Reference list

The references are listed in numerical order. Entries for journal articles, books, chapters in books, theses, and electronic media should have the following formats:

Entry in list for journal article   Authors' names, followed by initials with no full stops, separated by commas (if there are more than four authors, give the first three, followed by 'et al'), and followed by a full stop. Title of article, followed by full stop. Title of journal, or standard abbreviation, followed by date, semicolon, volume number, colon, page range, full stop. For abbreviations of journal titles, the Index Medicus system is nowadays almost universally used (see www.nlm.nih.gov/tsd/serials/lji.html). For example:

1. Baron DN. Ethical issues and clinical pathology. *J Clin Pathol* 1993; **46**: 385–7.
2. Kastelein JJP, van Leuven SI, Burgess L, et al, for the RADIANCE 1 Investigators. Effect of torcetrapib on carotid artery atherosclerosis in familial hypercholesterolemia. *N Engl J Med* 2007; **356**: 620–30.

Entry in list for book   Authors' names as for journal article. Title of book, followed by full stop. Place of publication, colon, publisher, comma, date, full stop. For example:

1. Baron DN, Whicher JT, Lee KE. *A New Short Textbook of Chemical Pathology,* 5th edn. London: Edward Arnold, 1989.

Entry in list for chapter in book   Authors' names as for journal article. Title of chapter, followed by full stop. 'In:', followed by editors' names (style as for authors' names), followed by 'eds' and full stop. Title of book, followed by full stop. Place of publication, colon, publisher, comma, date, colon, page range of chapter, full stop. For example:

1. Kipps TJ. The cluster of differentiation antigens. In: Beutler E, Lichtman MA, Coller BS, Kipps TJ, Seligsohn U, eds. *Williams Hematology,* 6th edn. New York: McGraw-Hill, 2001: 141–52.

Entry in list for thesis   A thesis should be quoted in the same way as for a book, and the name of the university must always be given so that the reader (theoretically) can consult the thesis.

Electronic media   References to non-paper sources are steadily increasing in frequency, and text superscript numbering should be used as for paper references. The list should give the appropriate website address (www. ..., etc.) and the last date on which the site was accessed.

Harvard system

This system was so called because it was first reported being used at Harvard University in 1881. The key feature is that authors' names are included in the text together with the date of publication. It is now less frequently used in journals (mainly for reasons of space).

In the text, the authors' names, without initials, are given, followed by the year (four or more authors should be cited as 'first author et al'): for example, '... Smith & Jones (1999) stated' or '... (Smith et al, 1999a)'. Electronic references that do not carry an author's name should be inserted in full in the text, without a separate entry in the list.

The list is arranged in alphabetical order of first authors' names, without numbering. For a given first author, entries should be in the following order: single-author papers by date; two-author papers alphabetically by second author; finally, multi-author papers by date (*not* by second author). If two or more entries by the same author(s) have the same date, they should be differentiated by adding a, b, etc. after the date. The structure of entries in the list is as for the Vancouver system, with the exception that the date (often in parentheses) should follow the authors' names. For example:

Baron DN (1993). Ethical issues and clinical pathology. *J Clin Pathol* **46**: 385–7.

Kipps TJ (2001). The cluster of differentiation antigens. In: Beutler E, Lichtman MA, Coller BS, Kipps TJ, Seligsohn U, eds. *Williams Hematology,* 6th edn. New York: McGraw-Hill: 2141–52.

Books

Here there is much more flexibility, with many publishers (especially if biomedical books are only a part of their output) having an idiosyncratic system with which prospective authors should familiarize themselves before completing the manuscript. The references may be in the same format as for journals, with a list either at the end of each chapter or collected at the end of the book, or they may be given as footnotes on each page. There may be a list of Further Reading for each chapter or for the whole book, without specific text referral. 'Further reading' and 'Bibliography' may be included with the references or as separate lists.

Theses

The Vancouver system is not recommended for theses, and the Harvard system should always be used.

The specific advantages of this system for theses are that it is then very much easier, when correcting and rewriting, to insert and remove references without the trouble of renumbering, as this carries a high probability of error. It is also much easier for the supervisor and examiners to check whether key references are included – especially to their own publications – without the need to check text numbers against the list.

Digital object identifiers

Digital object identifiers (DOIs/dois) are unique standardized (mainly numerical) article reference codes applicable to all published papers, whether online or in print on paper. It is the responsibility of the publisher, not of the author, to insert the appropriate DO1. A comparison for unique publication identifiers is the established ISBN system for books (and DOIs can equally be applied to books). The use of DOIs for reference is growing (a notable example being *Proceedings of the Royal Society*), but is by no means universal. When a journal article is published online before appearing in print, a DOI reference is provided before year/volume/page details are available.

A useful outline of the system is at www.doi.org and there is an excellent, more detailed description at www.uksg.org/serials/doi.asp.

4 | Proof correction marks

The following table gives a selection of the most commonly used proof correction marks, for the guidance of authors and editors, as recommended by British Standards. A full list of proof correction marks can be found in BS 5261-2:2005, available from BSI (British Standards Institution), 389 Chiswick High Road, London W4 4AL, UK.

Unless the journal or book publisher requires a different system, the following colour code should be used by authors and editors:

- typesetter's errors: red
- author's/editor's changes and comments: blue

(note that green marking should *not* be used – this colour is reserved for marks made by the typesetter).

General

Instructions	Mark in text	Mark in margin
End of change	None	/
Leave as is	Underline characters with ------	(√)
Remove superfluous marks	Circle marks to be removed	✕
Query accuracy with appropriate source	Circle affected words	(?)

Insertion, deletion, and replacement

Instructions	Mark in text	Mark in margin
Insert marginal material into body of text	⋀	Additional material followed by ⋀

Instructions	Mark in text	Mark in margin
Insert large quantity of additional text	λ	Letter in a diamond, followed by λ ⟨A⟩ λ Insertion on separate sheet (or in suitable area of white space on proof page), identified by ⟨A⟩
Delete	/ through single character ⊢——————⊣ through all characters or words to be deleted	⌒⌐
Delete and close up	∫ through single character ⊢————⊣ through all characters or words to be deleted	⌒⌐
Replace characters or words	/ through single character ⊢—————⊣ through all characters or or words to be replaced	Replacement character(s) words
Change font	Circle character(s) to be changed	⊗
Change to capital letters	Underline characters with ≡≡≡	≡≡
Change to small capital letters	Underline characters with ≡≡	≡
Change capital or small capital letters to lower case	Circle characters	$\not\equiv$, $\neq$
Change to italic type	Underline character(s) with ———	∠__/

Instructions	Mark in text	Mark in margin
Change to upright (roman) type	Circle character(s)	⌐⌐⌐
Change to bold type	Underline character(s) with ~~~~~	~~~
Change to non-bold type	Circle character(s)	~~~⌐~~~
Insert (or replace) character as inferior (subscript)	⋀ where character is to be inserted / through character to be replaced	over character, e.g. ⌐₂
Insert (or replace) character as superior (superscript)	⋀ where character is to be inserted / through character to be replaced	under character, e.g. ⁷₂
Insert (or replace by) full stop or decimal point	⋀ where required / through character to be replaced	⊙
Insert (or replace by) colon	⋀ where required / through character to be replaced	⊙
Insert (or replace by) semicolon	⋀ where required / through character to be replaced	;
Insert (or replace by) comma	⋀ where required / through character to be replaced	,
Insert (or replace by) apostrophe	⋀ where required / through character to be replaced	ˀ
Insert (or replace by) quotation marks	⋀ where required / through character to be replaced	⁇ or ⁇

Instructions	Mark in text	Mark in margin
Insert (or replace by) hyphen	$\wedge$ where required / through character to be replaced	⊢ − ⊣
Insert (or replace by) solidus	$\wedge$ where required / through character to be replaced	⊘
Insert underline	Circle character(s) or word(s)	⊜

Positioning

Instructions	Mark in text	Mark in margin
New paragraph		
Run on		
Transpose characters or words	or between characters or words (numbered if necessary for clarity)	or
Transpose lines	 (numbered if necessary)	
Centre	enclosing material to be centred	[ ]
Indent or shift to right		
Cancel indent or move to left		
Align right	enclosing material to be aligned right	

Instructions	Mark in text	Mark in margin
Align left	enclosing material to be aligned left	
Take over character(s), word(s), or line(s) to next line, column, or page		The mark surrounding the material to be taken over extends into the margin
Take back character(s), word(s), or line(s) to previous line, column, or page		The mark surrounding the material to be taken back extends into the margin
Shift material to position indicated	Enclose material to be shifted and indicate new position	
Raise material	above material to be raised below material to be raised	
Lower material	above material to be lowered below material to be lowered	
Correct vertical alignment		
Correct horizontal alignment		

Spacing

Instructions	Mark in text	Mark in margin
Delete space between characters or words (close up)	⌢ linking characters or ⌣ words	⌢ ⌣
Insert space between characters or words	|	⌄ If necessary, give the size of the space to be inserted
Reduce space between characters or words	|	⌃ If necessary, give the size to which the space is to be reduced
Equalize spacing between words in a line	| between affected words	⤥
Insert space between lines or paragraphs	⟶⟨ or ⟩⟶	The mark extends into the margin
Reduce space between lines or paragraphs	⟶⟩ or ⟨⟶	The mark extends into the margin

56